Doctor, WHY DOES DADDY SNORE?

From the *Doctor's Guide to Healthy Sleep Series*

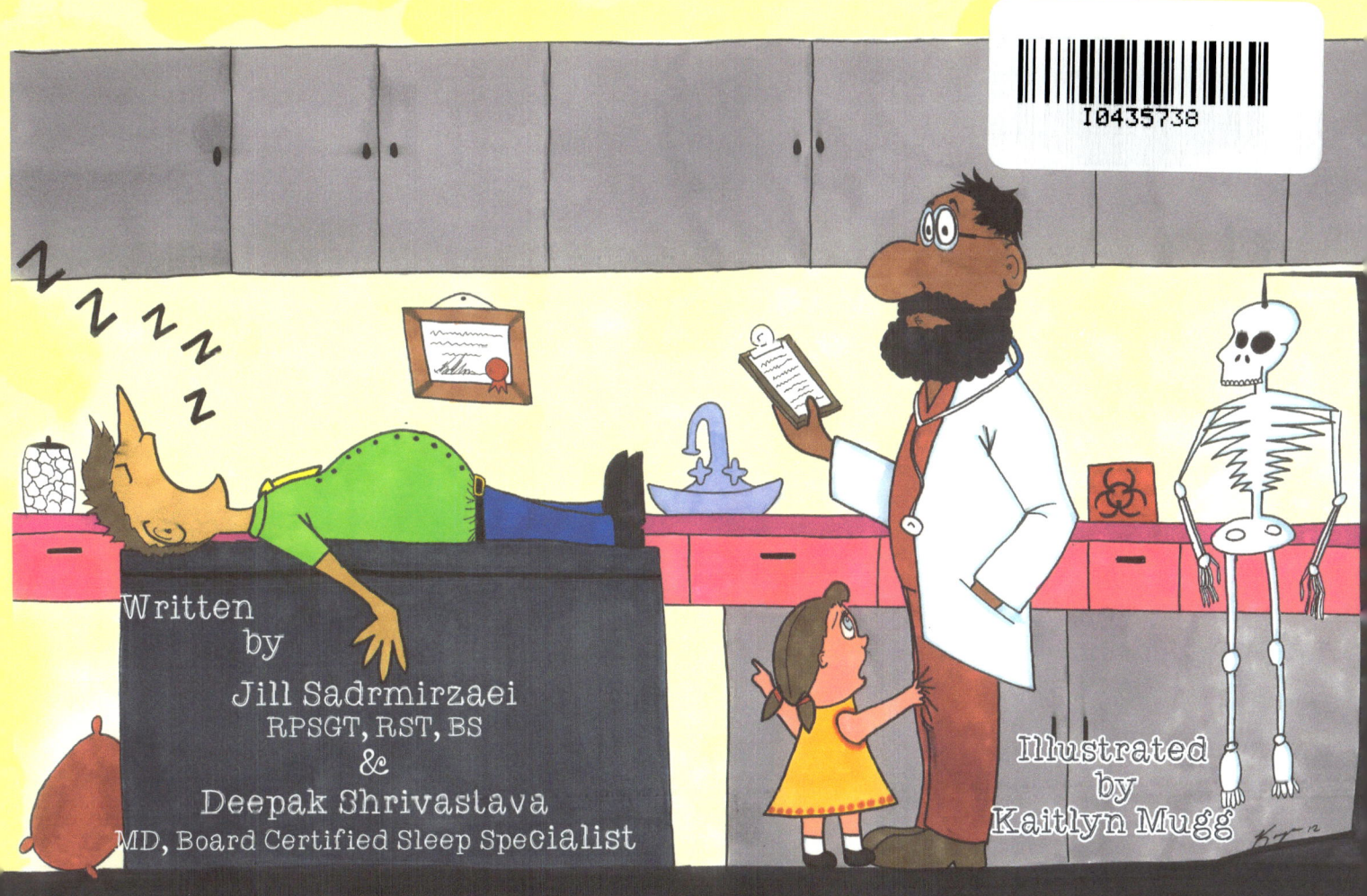

Written by
Jill Sadrmirzaei
RPSGT, RST, BS
&
Deepak Shrivastava
MD, Board Certified Sleep Specialist

Illustrated by
Kaitlyn Mugg

FOREWARD

Obstructive sleep apnea is a serious medical condition that is often overlooked and underdiagnosed. If untreated, it can lead to driving accidents, heart disease, stroke, diabetes, depression, and death. Obstructive sleep apnea can occur in all ages, but is most common in men and women in their middle ages. This is also the time when adults are in the prime of their lives, achieving success at work, and most importantly, growing their families.

Doctor, Why Does Daddy Snore, by Jill Sadrmirzaei and Dr. Deepak Shrivastava, serves a vital purpose. Anyone who has been around a young child knows how infinitely curious he or she can be. This book will help to satisfy the curiosity of children and to educate them and their families about snoring and obstructive sleep apnea, with the result of encouraging their family members and friends to be evaluated and treated by physicians specializing in sleep medicine.

Ms. Sadrmirzaei and Dr. Shrivastava should be congratulated in writing an outstanding book that will serve to educate children, parents, grandparents, and generations to come!

Clete A. Kushida, M.D., Ph.D., RPSGT
President, World Sleep Federation
Past President, American Academy of Sleep Medicine
Director, Stanford Sleep Medicine Center
Professor, Stanford University Medical Center

Acknowledgements

We would like to thank our patients who have contributed to our education and evolvement in sleep disorders. In addition, none of this would be possible without the unconditional support of our families: Kavita , Reza, Kim, and especially our children; Roopa Sirohi, MD, Aman ,Richa, Jordan, Mia, and Peyton whom constantly inspired us to continue our journey to change the generation!

> "Sleep is that golden chain that ties health and our bodies together."

Thomas Dekker

Peppard PE. Increased Prevalence of Sleep-Disordered Breathing in Adults. Am J Epidemiol. 2013 Apr.

Meir H. Kryger. Principles and practice of sleep medicine, 5th Edition

Flemons, W. W. "Clinical Practice: Obstructive Sleep Apnea." New England Journal of Medicine. 2002; 347:498–504.

Hoffstein, V. "Snoring." Chest 1996; 109: 201–222.

©2011 Jill Sadrmirzaei, Deepak Shrivastava

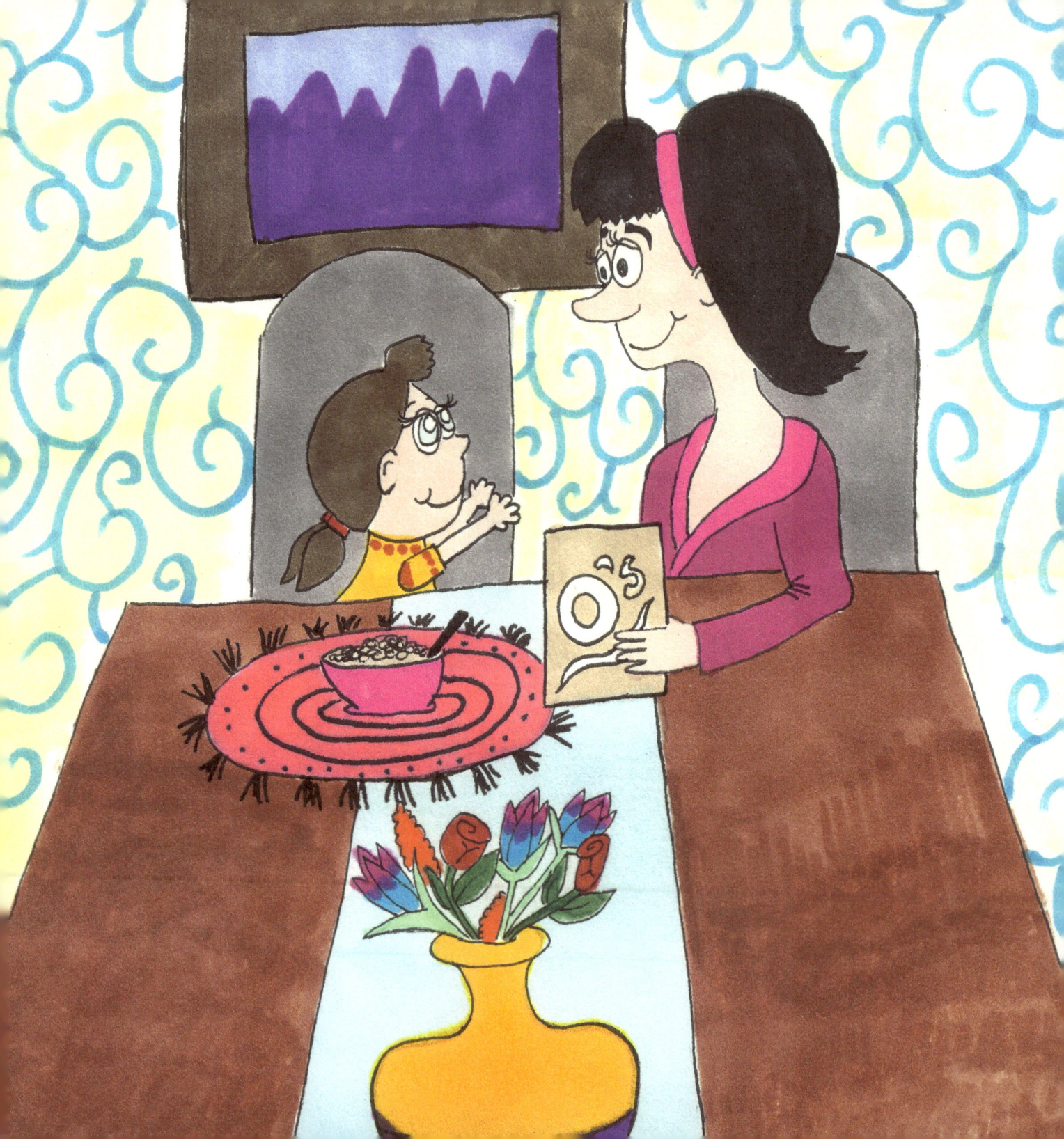

This is a great morning! Mommy and I are going to see Doctor D. I like Doctor D. He always says hello to me, and his receptionist (a big word meaning the lady who sits at the front desk) always gives me stickers and snacks.

I am very excited about this visit to Doctor D's office because Daddy is going too. He never goes to the doctor with us. Daddy is never sick and never needs shots.

"Is Daddy OK?" I said to Mommy this morning.

"Of course he is," said Mommy. "He just has some questions for Doctor D about his sleep."

I am very curious (a neat word meaning interested) about our visit, so during breakfast I ask Daddy the big question that I could not wait to ask this morning.

"Daddy, why are you going with us to Doctor D's? Do you need a shot?" Daddy is reading his paper, so I ask again. "Daddy, why are you coming with us?"

"Well, sweetie, Daddy snores," Mommy says. She is looking at Daddy with her eyebrow all funny when she says this.

"I like it when you snore, Daddy. You sound like a bear at the zoo." Why does Doctor D want to hear Daddy snore? "Ohhh," I say. "Doctor D wants to play zoo animals with us?" Daddy can be the bear and Doctor D can be the lion.

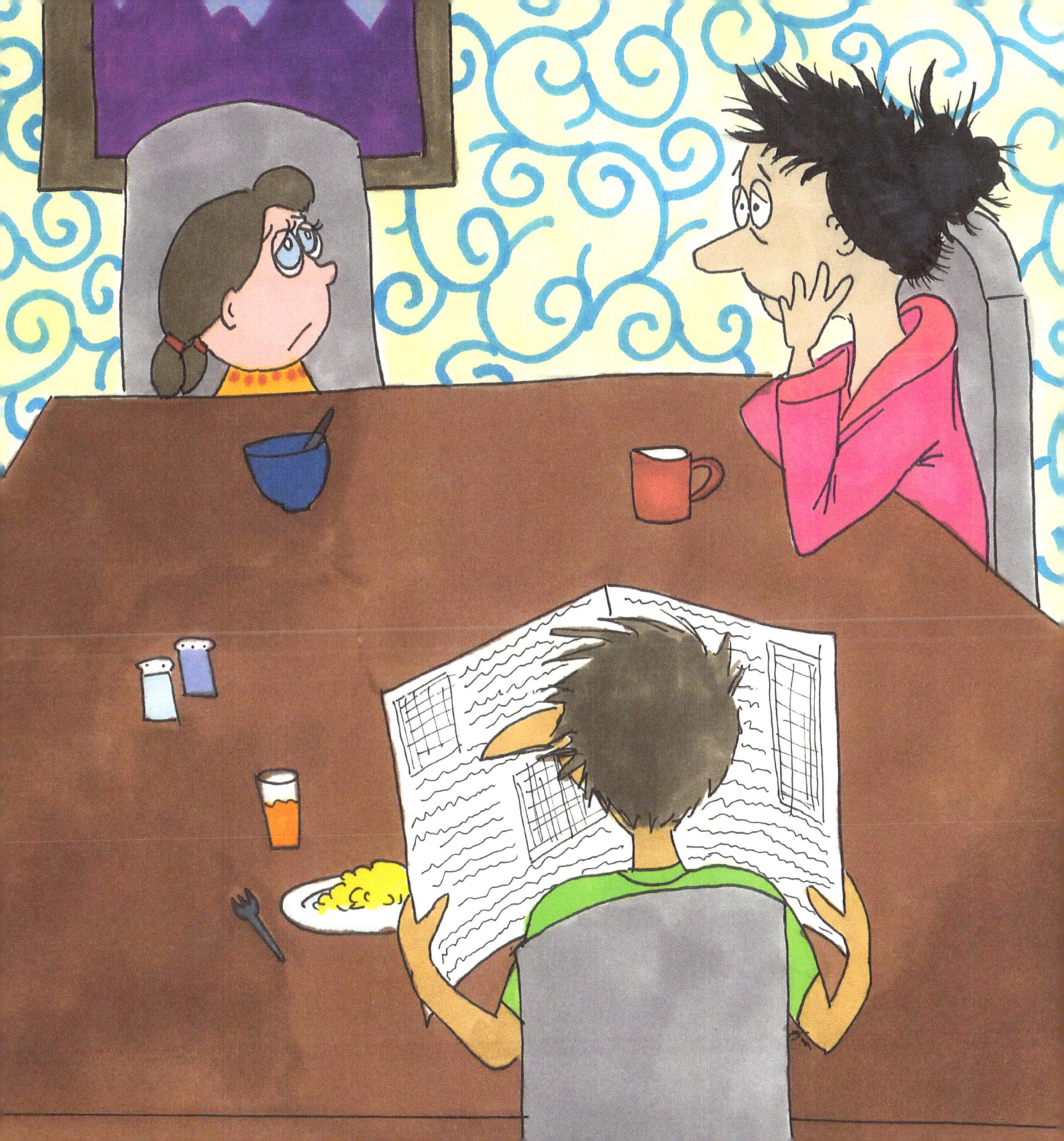

"I am sure we would all have fun playing pretend zoo animals, Mia, but I am tired during the day, and I wake up your mom at night," Daddy says. "That's why I need to see Doctor D."

Mommy looks at Daddy with her eyebrow all funny again when he says this, and then she says, "I haven't slept well in months."

Wow. I think Doctor D has a lot of work to do. I am still not sure why funny noises and being tired are reasons to see Doctor D, but I am eager to find out. "Whatever it is, Daddy, Doctor D will have a shot for it," I say.

"Thanks, Mia. I hope I do not need any shots."

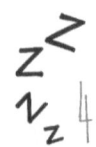

4

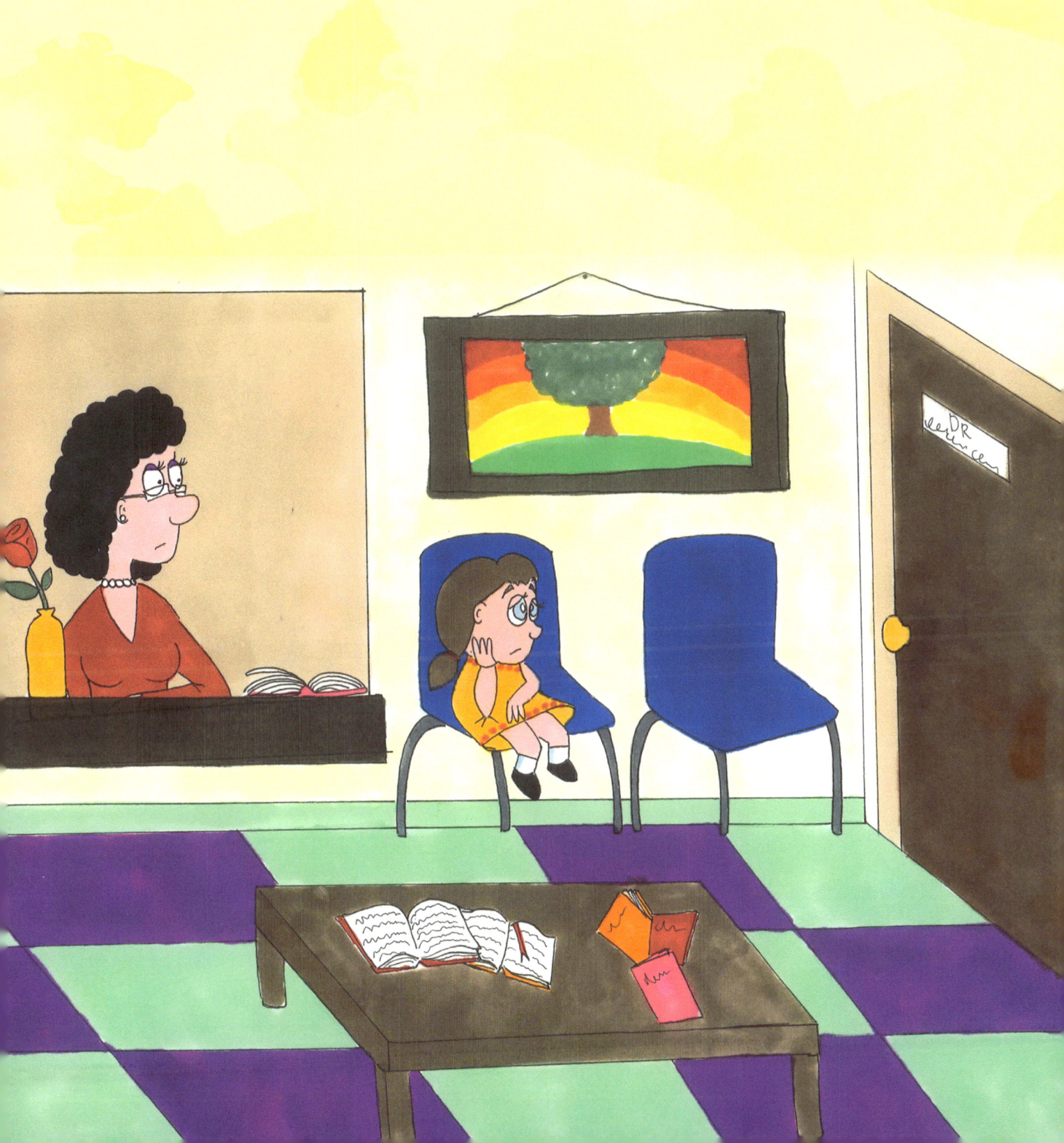

We got in the car and went to Doctor D's office; Pam the receptionist said "Is your dad ready to see Doctor D?"

"Sure thing," I say, "but I am still curious about why we came to see Doctor D for his snoring."

"Well, Mia," Pam says, "Doctor D specializes (an important word meaning studied for years) in sleep medicine. Your dad may have a sleep disorder. A disorder refers to a function of the body that doesn't work right. All that noise your dad is making at night is a sign that something could be wrong with his sleep and his breathing."

> Dr. D says:
> The prevalence in the United States is estimated to be 10% for 30-49-year-old men; 17% of 50-70-year-old men; 3% for 30-49-year-old women; and 9% of 50-70 year-old women. It varies with race and gender.
> For example, African Americans and Asians have a higher prevalence of the disorder compared with other ethnic groups.

Wow, I think, sleep is more difficult than I thought. They even have doctors for it!

z
z
z
z 6

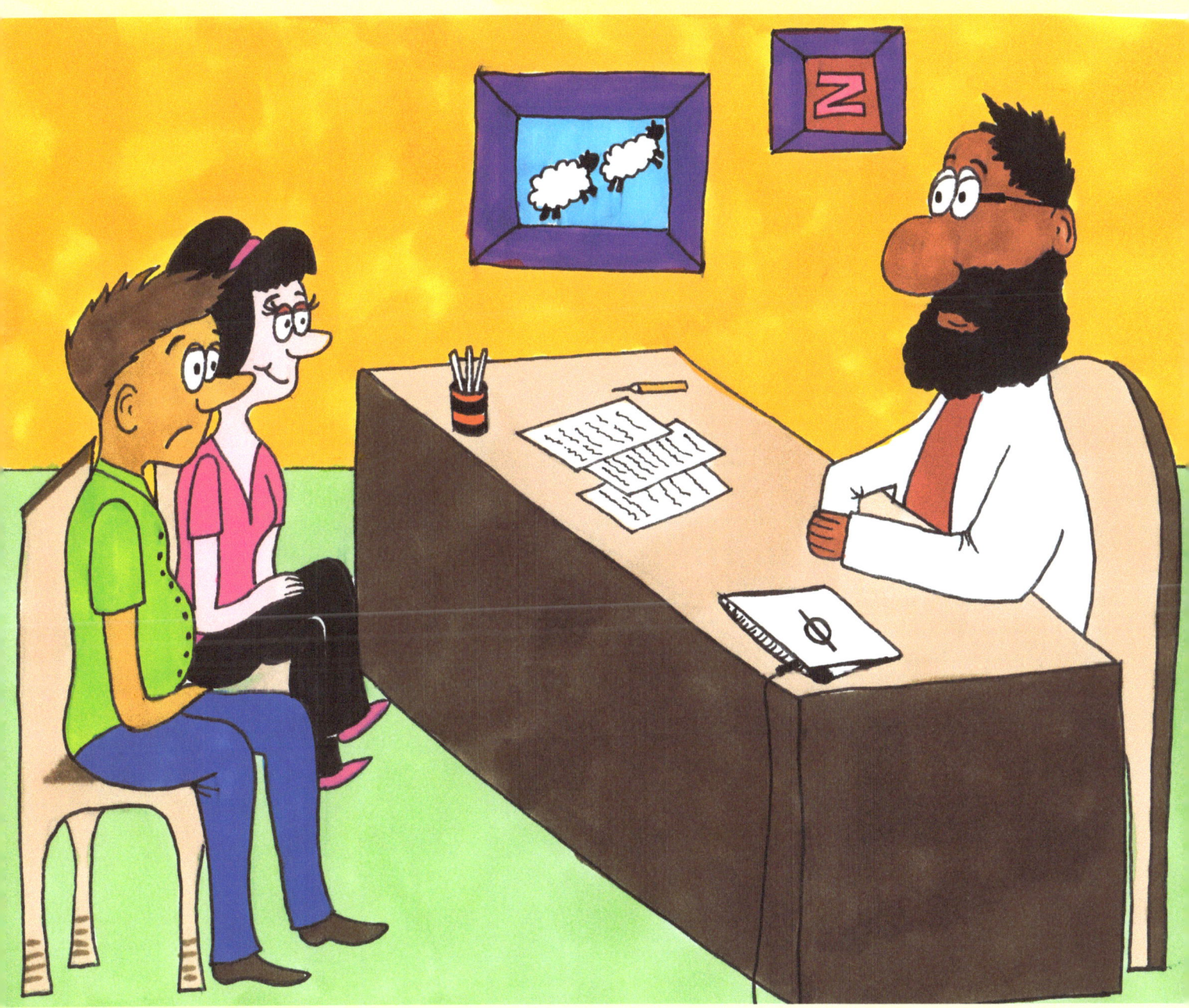

Just then Doctor D walks out to get Mommy and Daddy. "Hi, Mia," he says.

"Hi, Doctor D, can you help my daddy with his sleep?"

"I can certainly try, Mia. Why don't I talk to your mom and dad in my office, and I will speak with you after we are done," he says. "Pam, will you take Mia to the playroom?"

"Ohhh...cool, Doctor D! I love this part of my visit. I can't wait to watch videos and play with the toys."

Dr. D says:
The most common symptom of sleep apnea is snoring. Other common complaints are choking, gasping, cessation of breathing, morning headaches, and nocturnal urination. Many patients report excessive daytime sleepiness. Some people report fatigue, impaired intellectual performance, and even mood and behavior problems. In children, hyperactivity and poor school performance are commonly noted. If left undiagnosed or untreated, sleep apnea can be associated with high blood pressure, heart attack, and stroke.
Sleep apnea can be easily confirmed with a sleep study, also known as a polysomnogram.

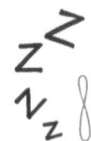

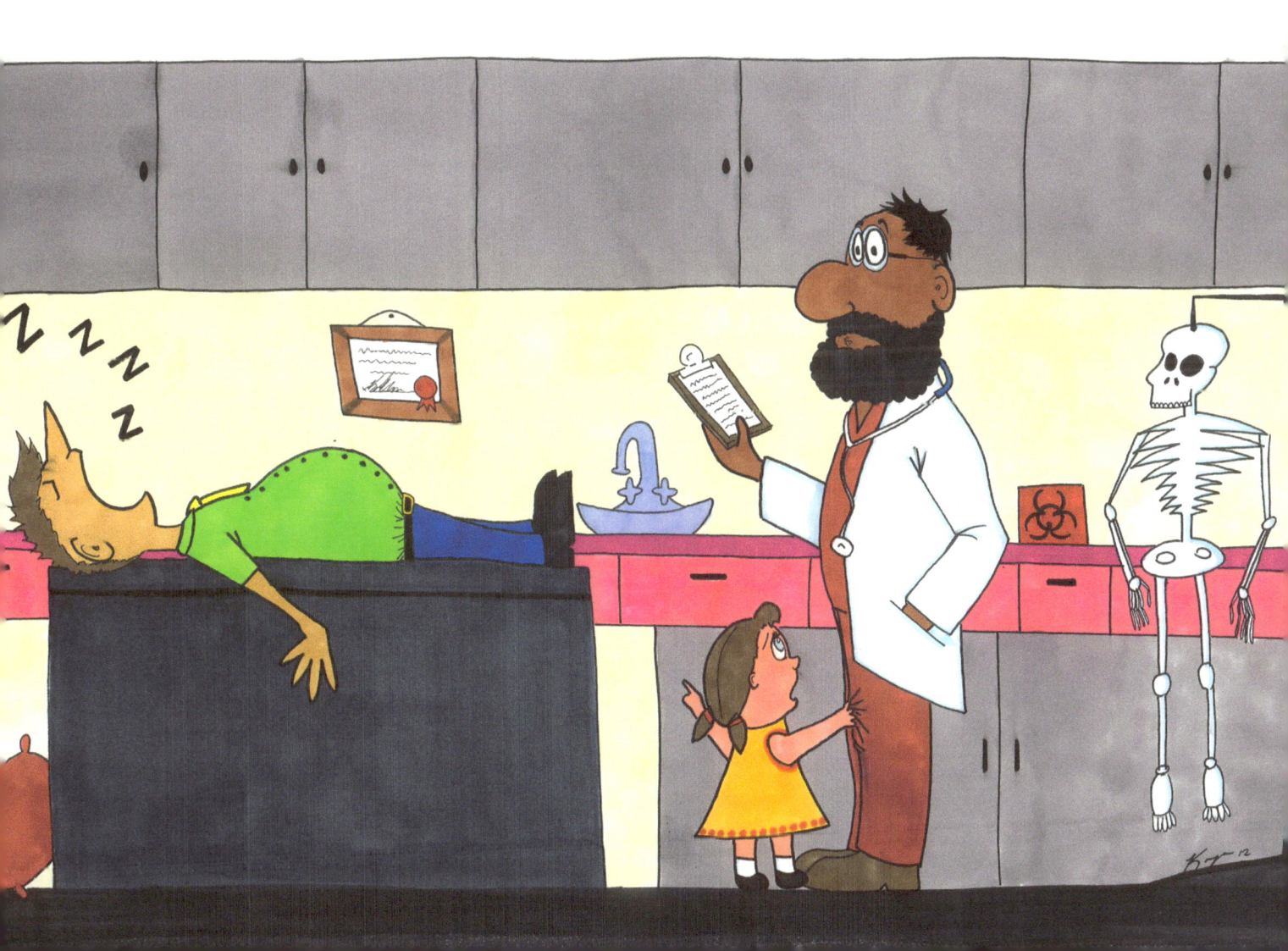

A short time later, Pam takes me to Doctor D's office to talk with Mommy and Daddy.

"Mia," he says, "your dad is snoring at night, and it may be unhealthy (meaning not well) for him. I have discussed this with your mom and dad, and they have agreed that your dad should come back to our office for overnight testing. Do you have any questions?"

"Wow, Doctor D," I say. "What if my daddy doesn't pass the sleep test? Will he have to go to sleep school?"

Dr. D says:
A sleep study is a pain-free test done overnight in a comfortable facility called a sleep lab. A number of wires are secured by sticky tape on the patient's head, chin, chest, and leg to record the body's electrical signals during sleep. Small cannulas (plastic sensors) are placed in front of the nose and mouth to record the flow of air in and out, and one belt each is placed on the chest and abdomen to record the movements of these areas with the breathing. A probe is placed on a finger to record oxygen levels in the blood. Patients are still able to sleep comfortably despite all of these wires and belts! A technician is present throughout the night to make sure all of the wires stay in place and the data is recorded.

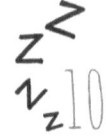

10

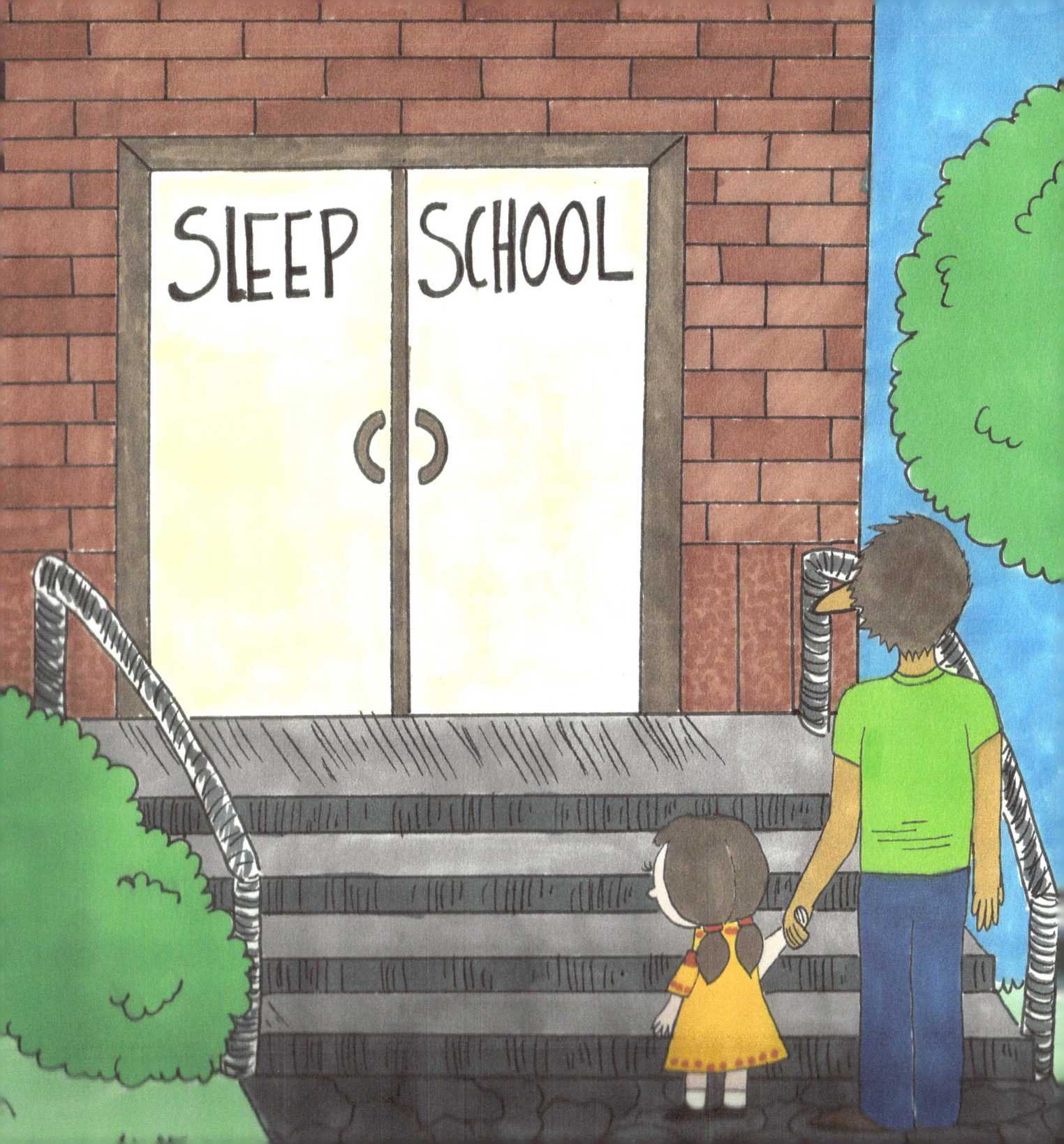

"Not exactly, Mia. The test is used to find out if your dad has any physiological (a Greek word meaning a part of our body) problems that may be disturbing his sleep at night."

Dr. D says:
Sometimes a sleep study can be done at a patient's home. There is no technician to monitor the test at home. The test has fewer wires and is less comprehensive. A doctor will determine what the best method is for the patient.

"I am not sure if I understand all this," I say. "Doctor D, you are not going to hurt Daddy, are you?"

"Oh no, Mia, the test is easy. We put some things on your dad that look like Band-Aids, and then he goes to sleep in a bed alone. How does that sound?"

"OK, I guess. Daddy, will you be OK?"

"Of course," Daddy says. "It will be fun. I love to sleep."

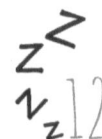

12

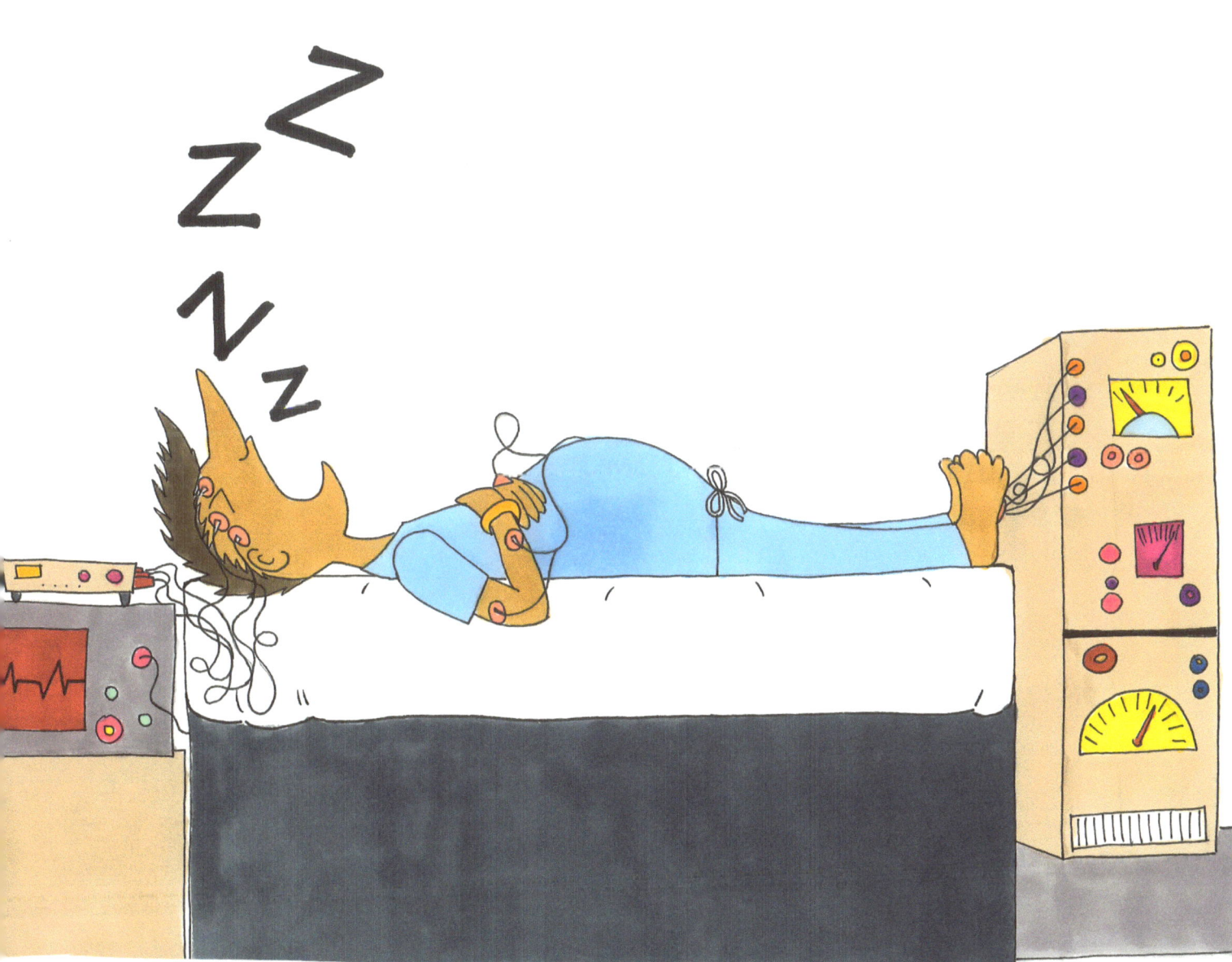

"But Doctor D, what if Daddy doesn't pass his test? Will he get a bad report card in sleeping?"

"Oh no, Mia. We will then have to treat your father at night. A treatment is something that helps your dad. There are several treatments we can use." "He will then get a good grade on his health card."

Dr. D says:
There are many options for treating sleep apnea. Weight loss, positional therapy, and some medications may be considered to treat snoring and mild forms of sleep apnea. However, the most efficacious and recommended treatment is using a mask over the nose, which is attached to a machine with tubing. The machine, called a PAP (positive airway pressure) machine, blows air through the back of the throat to keep it from collapsing. Milder forms of sleep apnea can be treated with specially made dental devices called oral appliances. In addition, the airway can be opened up by surgical operation. Every option has its own advantages.

"Oh great, Doctor D! Then will Daddy stop making that noise?"

"He sure will, Mia. Then your mom and dad will both sleep better."

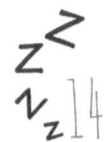

14

A week later Daddy's test results were completed and Dr. D recommended he begins using the PAP treatment (a cool medical word meaning a device that helps him) while he sleeps. Now, every morning when Mommy makes breakfast, she says how good it was to sleep without Daddy's snoring. Daddy seems rested and happier, too. I think that Doctor D is a genius (meaning very smart). I did not know that sleep was so important for our health.

THE END

z Z
z
z z 15

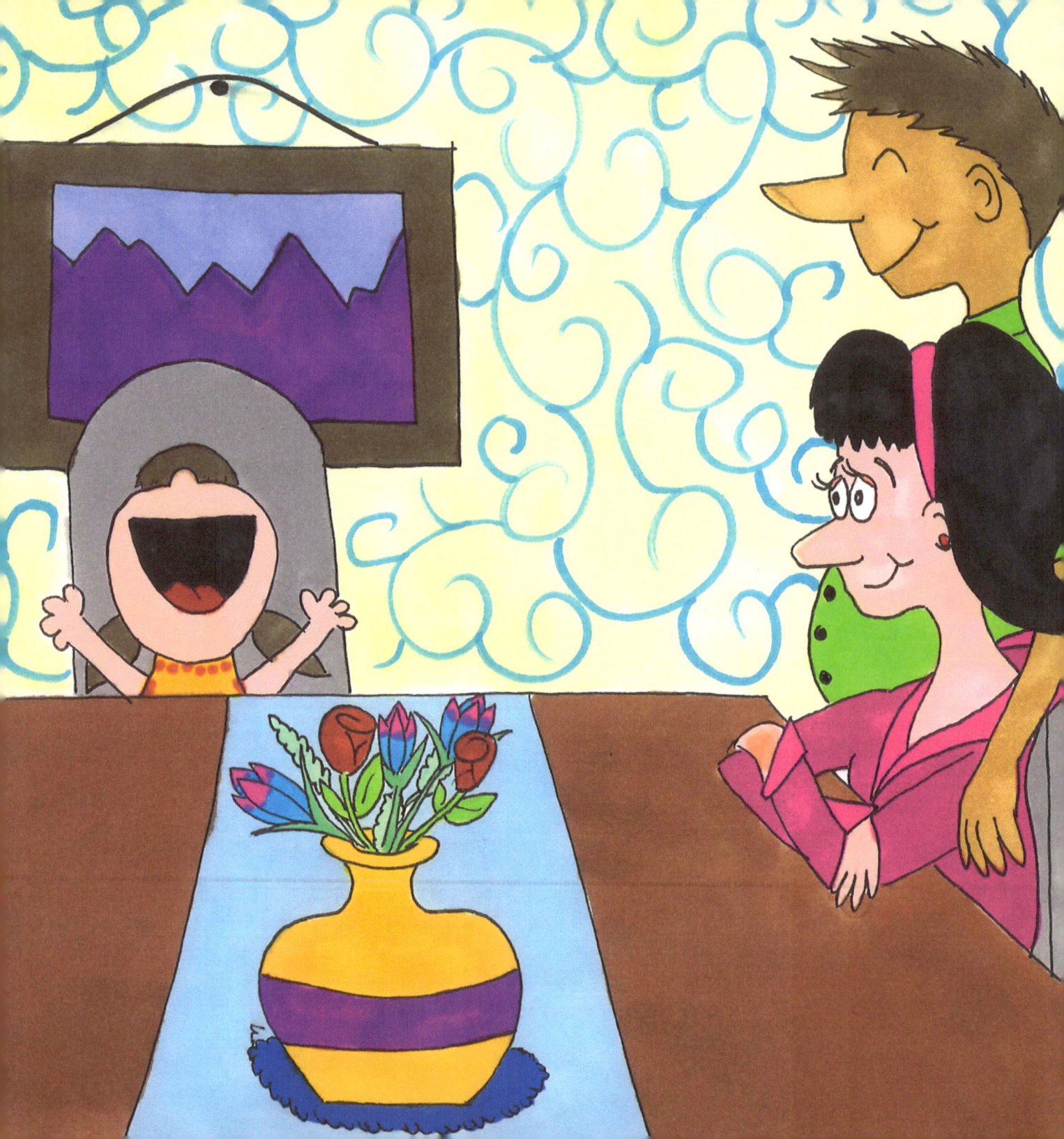

ABOUT THE AUTHORS

Deepak Shrivastava, MD brings extensive knowledge and expertise to the series of children's books. He received his Sleep Medicine training at Stanford and is board certified in Sleep Medicine, Pulmonary Medicine, Critical Care Medicine, and Internal Medicine.

Currently, he is a professor at UC Davis School of Medicine, and is the director of San Joaquin General Hospital Sleep Diagnostics Center.

He is recipient of many academic awards. His teaching efforts are known around the world. Dr. Shrivastava is a recognized icon in sleep communities in the global marketplace.

Dr. Shrivastava enjoys reading, music, tennis, and occasionally just not doing anything.

Jill Sadrmirzaei, RPSGT, RST, BS has been involved in promoting the cause of sleep medicine and providing education for over twenty years. She obtained her RPSGT in 1998. She was awarded the certificate of a Clinical Sleep Educator by the BRPT in 2013 and currently provides instruction in Polysomnography at collegiate institutions. She is also the National Clinical Manager of the sleep division at a corporation that provides sleep diagnostics services.

Jill enjoys reading, music, napping, spending time with her three children, and cultural/social activism.

Sleep Medicine Resources

Educational information for your friends and family can be found at the following websites:

Sleep Education: www.Sleepcenters.org

National Sleep Foundation http://sleepfoundation.org/

American Academy of Sleep Medicine http://www.aasmnet.org

World Sleep Federation http://worldsleepfederation.org/

American Sleep Apnea Association http://www.sleepapnea.org/

American academy of Dental Sleep Medicine http://www.aadsm.org/